Table of Contents

Overview

Scope and Purpose of These Guidelines

The subject matter in this document applies to all personnel working in the BOP Dental Service. All BOP facilities are encouraged to follow this program in the dental treatment of their inmates.

This document establishes guidelines for identifying and managing oral disease risks in the Federal Bureau of Prisons (BOP) Health Care System. The BOP *Clinical Practice Guidelines for Preventive Dentistry* represent a collation of acceptable practices for the dental management and treatment of oral conditions, including dental caries, periodontal disease, and oral cancer. Early detection of disease and intervention can significantly improve the oral health and well-being of inmate patients.

These guidelines provide a framework for the delivery of quality oral healthcare/preventive services, and to sustain continuous improvement of dental practice in the BOP. They are not intended to restrict individual clinical judgment.

Focus on Prevention

Modern methodology for the prevention of progressive oral diseases includes the identification of patients at high risk of developing diseases. These individuals are distinguished by demographics, lifestyles, and other risk indicators associated with the diseases.

Prevention is the most cost-effective means of controlling oral diseases and improving oral health among the BOP inmate population. Standardization of risk management protocols helps to direct appropriate treatment, based on risk levels.

These guidelines are complementary to the American Dental Association (ADA) Clinical Practice Parameters, applicable sections of the ADA Principles of Ethics and Code of Professional Conduct, and other nationally recognized guidelines cited in this document. The most recent versions of cited professional guidelines take precedence over previously published editions. Providers and clinical quality managers should be knowledgeable about these and other pertinent guidelines, and should use them to develop effective programs to ensure quality care and the safety and health of patients and dental personnel.

The treatment protocols, based on the best available evidence, are intended to help guide treatment decisions regarding diagnosis, management, and treatment of oral diseases, including dental caries, periodontal disease, and oral cancer. Implementation of these treatment guidelines is encouraged, based upon availability of resources, patients' compliance, and providers' professional expertise and clinical judgment.

Evidence-Based Dentistry (EBD)

Evidenced-Based Dentistry forms the basis of clinical practice in the BOP Dental Service. The ADA (ADA Council on Scientific Affairs, 2006) defines the term "evidence-based dentistry" as follows: *EBD is an approach to oral health care that requires the judicious integration of systematic assessments of clinically relevant scientific evidence, relating to the patient's oral and medical condition and history, with the dentist's clinical expertise and the patient's treatment needs and preferences.*

Dental Caries

1. Tooth Decay: A Chronic Disease

Tooth decay (dental caries) is one of the most prevalent chronic diseases of people worldwide; individuals are susceptible to this disease throughout their lifetimes. A study published in 2005 found that 90% of adults had dental caries in their permanent teeth, and 23% had untreated tooth decay (Beltrán-Aguilar, et al., 2005).

Tooth mineral is normally lost and gained in a continuous process of deminerlization and remineralization. Dental caries is a disease of the hard tissues of the tooth, occurring when the demineralization, caused by cariogenic bacteria, exceeds remineralization. Over time, dental caries forms through a complex interaction between acid-producing bacteria and fermentable carbohydrate, influenced by many host factors including condition of the teeth and saliva flow. The disease affects both the crowns and roots of teeth, and it can arise in early childhood as an aggressive form of tooth decay that affects the primary teeth of children.

Initially, caries appears as white spots. Active caries appears as rough, opaque spots, while inactive caries is hard and appears shiny. Active caries progresses from decalcified spots to cavitation. If left untreated, the disease progresses to pain, infection, and eventual tooth loss.

2. Topical Fluoride as Preventative Therapy

Dentistry has increasingly incorporated the medical mode of treatment, turning to pharmacological agents to arrest and reverse the disease process, instead of relying solely on surgical interventions (as in the past) to repair dentition after the disease has taken its toll. Presently, several methods are employed for the prevention and remineralization of caries, including the application of fluoride, chlorhexidine (CHX), xylitol, and casein phosphopeptide-amorphous calcium phosphate (CPP-ACP).

→ *The protocols in these guidelines promote the application of topical fluoride therapy since there is consistent and strong evidence of its effectiveness, based on a sizable body of evidence from randomized controlled trials.*

Fluoride is a mineral that helps prevent tooth decay by enhancing remineralization of affected (demineralized) enamel, converting the tooth's calcium mineral apatite into fluorapatite, which makes tooth enamel more resistant to bacteria-generated acid attacks. Fluoride treatment has been the mainstay of caries prevention therapy since the introduction of water fluoridation over six decades ago (Grand Rapids, Michigan, was fluoridated in 1945). Fluoride helps to control the initiation and progression of caries. The effect of fluoride is largely topical. Different modes of fluoride applications are available, including fluoride dentifrices (toothpastes), gels, mouth rinses, and varnishes.

Research on Fluoride's Effectiveness

Systematic reviews and meta-analyses of fluoride treatment for caries prevention (predominantly on children and adolescents) show that:

- **Fluoride toothpaste concentrations of 1000 ppm or above are significantly better than placebo.** There is some evidence of a dose-dependent effect, i.e., the higher the fluoride concentration, the greater the effectiveness, but the differences were not always statistically significant. (Walsh, et al., 2010)

- **Fluoride toothpastes appear to be similar to mouth rinses and gels in effectiveness.** The data comparing varnishes to mouth rinses and gels found that fluoride toothpastes, mouth rinses, and gels reduce tooth decay in children and adolescents to a similar extent. Nevertheless, toothpastes are more likely to be regularly used. (Marinho, et al., 2004b)

- **The benefits of combination regimens are unclear.** The meta-analysis of the nine studies assessing the effect of fluoride mouth rinses, gels, or varnishes used in combination with fluoride toothpaste on the permanent dentition indicates that their combined use is associated with a reduction in decayed, missing, and filled tooth surfaces. However, the average reduction of 10% was not substantial. (Marinho, et al., 2004a)

- **Periodic, professionally applied fluoride is recommended for some patients.** Evidence-based clinical recommendations for professionally-applied fluoride in caries prevention, among moderate- and high-risk adults, call for the application of fluoride gel or varnish every 3 to 6 months, depending on the caries risk levels. Low-risk adults may not receive additional benefit from professional topical fluoride application; fluoridated water and fluoride toothpastes may provide adequate caries prevention in this risk category. (ADA Council on Scientific Affairs, 2006)

- **Existing strategies for caries prevention are also likely to be effective for arresting and reversing early caries lesions.** Strategies for primary prevention and remineralization include topical application of fluorides. The research data on fluorides in water and dentifrices support their efficacy. The data also supports the use of fluoride varnishes. (NIH Consensus Development Panel, 2001)

- **Fluoride reduces caries in people of all ages and is effective and safe when used correctly.** The correct use of fluoride has been said to have dramatically reduced tooth decay over the past few decades. Fluoride toothpaste, if used as recommended, is safe to use irrespective of low, normal, or high fluoride exposure from other sources. The recommended fluoride concentration in toothpaste for permanent dentition is 1000–1500 ppm fluoride, with a minimum of 800 ppm F bioavailable. Additional use of fluoride mouth rinses may be indicated for individuals at risk of developing caries: both daily rinsing with 0.05% NaF (226 ppm F) and once-a-week or once-every-two-weeks rinsing with 0.2% NaF (909 ppm F) were found to be effective. (Zero, Marinho, Phantumvanit, 2012)

Types of Fluoride (F)

Sodium Fluoride (NaF):

- Most over-the-counter toothpastes contain 0.243% NaF (equivalent to 1105 ppm F), while prescription-strength toothpaste contains 1.1% NaF (equivalent to 5000 ppm F).

- Most gels are 2% NaF (equivalent to 9050 ppm F or 0.9% F), while varnishes typically contain 5% NaF (equivalent to 22600 ppm F or 2.26% F).

- NaF is also available as mouth rinses in 0.2% and 0.05% concentrations for weekly and daily use, respectively.

- Use of NaF is recommended for patients with any type of restorative material, including porcelain restorations.

Acidulated Phosphate Fluoride (APF):

- APF is formulated to increase enamel's uptake of F in the acidic environment; it has a pH of 3. It is found in gels and mouth rinses, as well as in prophylaxis pastes.

- Gels and prophylaxis pastes contain 1.23% APF, which is equivalent to 12300 ppm F. Mouth rinses are available in 0.022% F concentrations for daily use.

- APF formulations are not recommended for patients with porcelain restorations as APF may affect the smoothness and gloss of the porcelain surface.

Stannous Fluoride (SnF_2):

- SnF_2 is used in toothpastes, rinses, and gels. Toothpastes contain 0.4% SnF_2, or 966 ppm F.

- It has been shown that SnF_2 is more effective than NaF in controlling gingivitis and gingival bleeding. It is one of the active ingredients in Crest Pro-Health toothpaste.

- SnF_2 formulations may cause temporary staining of teeth and restorations, which can be removed during prophylaxis procedures.

Sodium Monofluorophosphate Fluoride (MFP):

- MFP is used in toothpastes in concentrations of 0.76% MFP or around 1000 ppm F.

3. Dental Caries Risk Assessment

Caries risk assessment includes evaluation of physical, biological, environmental, behavioral, and lifestyle-related indicators such as high numbers of cariogenic bacteria, inadequate salivary flow, insufficient fluoride exposure, poor oral hygiene, cariogenic diet, and low socioeconomic status. *However, the most consistent predictor of caries risk is past caries experience* (Nevelle, 2009).

The approach to primary prevention should be based on common risk indicators. Secondary prevention and treatment should focus on the management of the caries process over time for individual patients, with a minimally invasive, tissue-preserving approach.

The provider may perform a caries risk assessment on inmates presenting to the clinic with multiple carious lesions. This can be conducted during the initial Admission and Orientation Examination (A&O Exam) and/or subsequent Comprehensive and Periodic oral examinations. Patients are classified as at low-, moderate-, or high-risk for future caries. Risk level assignment is based on the professional expertise and clinical judgment of the practitioner.

→ *Table 1* below lists risk criteria for dental caries. *Table 2* lists the BOP protocol for risk management of dental caries. (The information in these tables is adapted from the *Oral Disease Risk Management Protocols in the Navy Military Health System*, BUMEDINST 6600.16A, August 23, 2010.)

Table 1. Risk Criteria for Dental Caries

Low Risk	Moderate Risk	High Risk
1. *No carious lesions during current exam* – no cavitations or active decay. Patients with inactive or arrested lesions are at lower risk. *or* 2. *No factors that may increase caries risk significantly, including:* • Poor oral hygiene • Cariogenic diet • Presence of exposed root surfaces • Enamel defects or genetic abnormality of teeth • Many multi-surface restorations • Restoration overhangs or open margins • Active orthodontic treatment • Chemotherapy or radiation therapy • Eating disorders • Physical or mental disability with inability to perform proper oral health care	1. *One or two carious lesions during current exam* – cavitations or active decay. *or* 2. *No carious lesions during current exam, but presence of at least one factor* that may increase caries risk significantly (see bulleted list in "Low Risk" column).	1. *Three or more carious lesions during current exam* – cavitations or active decay. *or* 2. *Presence of multiple factors* that may increase caries risk significantly (see bulleted list in "Low Risk" column). *and/or* 3. *Xerostomia* – Drug-, radiation-, or disease-induced xerostomia is in itself a significant risk factor. *and/or* 4. *New carious lesion(s)* – Past caries experience is the best predictor for future caries.

Table 2. BOP Protocol for Dental Caries Risk Management

	Low Risk for Caries*	Moderate Risk for Caries	High Risk for Caries**

Protocol	1. Oral hygiene instruction.
	2. Fluoride dentifrice.
	
	* *A patient with Low-Risk Caries status for years does not require intervention or modification of OH practices.*
		1. Oral hygiene instruction.
		2. Fluoride dentifrice.
		3. Caries control:
		  a. Restore cavitated lesions.
		  b. Apply sealants for pits and fissures at risk.
		  c. Remineralize early non-cavitated lesions
		4. Dietary counseling.
		5. F mouth rinses, and varnish or fluoride gel applications.
			1. Oral hygiene instruction.
			2. Fluoride dentifrice.
			3. Caries elimination:
			  a. Restore cavitated lesions.
			  b. Apply sealants for pits and fissures.
			  c. Remineralize early non-cavitated lesions
			4. Dietary counseling.
			5. F mouth rinses, and varnish or fluoride gel applications.
			6. Evaluation of salivary flow (review meds & med hx).
			
			** *See Section 4, Treatment Protocol for Patients at High Risk for Caries, below.*

Recall	One Year	6–12 Months	3–6 months

4. Treatment Protocol for Patients at High Risk for Dental Caries

Strategies for caries prevention are also likely to be effective for arresting and reversing early carious lesions (NIH Consensus Development Panel, 2001). The three components of the BOP treatment protocol for high-risk patients are discussed below: ***Patient Education***, ***Treatment***, and ***Documentation*** (adapted from the *Oral Disease Risk Management Protocols in the Navy Military Health System*, BUMEDINST 6600.16A, August 23, 2010).

Patient Education

1) **Inform the patient that carious lesions are not the disease**, but the result of a disease process caused by high bacterial levels in his or her mouth. While placing a filling restores the damaged tooth, it may have little effect on the disease itself.

   → *Therefore, in addition to tooth restoration, dental caries treatment must address the cause of the bacterial build-up.*

2) **Inform the patient that he/she will be receiving antibacterial treatment** designed to control the bacteria in his or her mouth.

   → *Success will depend largely on their following the prescribed treatment.*

Treatment

1) **Eliminate active caries.**

   a) Restore any cavitated lesions. Glass ionomer-based restorative materials over resin composites are reasonable materials of choice on dentin and cementum because they chemically bond, have less shrinkage, release fluoride, and are biocompatible. Preps should be dried, but not desiccated (Jenson, et al., 2007).

   b) Seal the deep, retentive pits and fissures at risk.

2) **Implement preventive and remineralizing measures** (may be completed concurrently with elimination of active caries).

   a) Conduct a diet survey and modification.

   b) Provide oral health instruction (disease etiology and oral hygiene instruction).

   - Provide fluoride treatment using either varnishes or gels as per current professional guidelines. Fluoride varnish is normally applied twice a year. Studies show efficacy for applications ranging from 2 to 4 times a year. Varnish could be applied after patients have brushed their teeth; a dental prophylaxis is not necessary prior to application (Beltrán-Aguilar, et al., 2000; Marinho, et al., 2002).

   - Fluoride gel is recommended 2 to 4 times a year. Application time should be 4 minutes (ADA Council on Scientific Affairs, 2006).

   c) Very weak evidence and nonsignificant results exist in support of the use of CHX and CPP-ACP (Rethman MP, et al., ADA Council on Scientific Affairs, 2011).

3) **Schedule recall appointments.**

   a) Monitor and reinforce preventive measures.

   b) Monitor risk factors for appropriate therapy.

Documentation

All preventive instructions and treatment rendered will be documented in the Dental Treatment Notes (progress notes) of the dental portion of the Bureau Electronic Health Record (BEMR).

Periodontal Disease

1. Periodontal Terminology

Periodontium: The tissues that surround and support the teeth, including the gums, periodontal ligament, and bone.

Periodontics: The branch of dentistry that specializes in treating the supporting tissues of the teeth and in the placement, maintenance, and treatment of *dental implants*.

Periodontal disease: For the purposes of epidemiological research, *periodontal disease* is defined very specifically.

- **For a person to have periodontal disease**, he or she must have at least one periodontal site with 3 millimeters or more of attachment loss and 4 millimeters or more of pocket depth.
- **Moderate periodontal disease** is defined as having at least two teeth with interproximal attachment loss of 4 millimeters or more **or** at least two teeth with 5 millimeters or more of pocket depth at interproximal sites.
- **Severe periodontal disease** is defined as having at least two teeth with interproximal attachment loss of 6 millimeters or more **and** at least one tooth with 5 millimeters or more of pocket depth at interproximal sites.

Periodontitis: Periodontal disease involving bone loss around the teeth.

Chronic periodontitis: A form of periodontal disease characterized by inflammation within the supporting tissues of the teeth, progressive attachment loss and bone loss, and pocket formation and/or recession of the gingiva. Chronic periodontitis is recognized as the most frequently occurring form of periodontal disease. It is prevalent in adults, but can occur at any age. Progression of attachment loss usually occurs slowly, but periods of rapid progression can occur.

Periodontitis as a manifestation of systemic diseases: Periodontitis, often with onset at a young age, is associated with one of several systemic diseases, such as diabetes.

Other periodontal terms:

Abscess: Localized collection of pus in a space formed by the disintegration of tissues; may be either gingival or periodontal in nature.

Calculus (tartar): Hardened *dental plaque*. Calculus is usually hard, rough, and porous.

Dental plaque: A sticky, colorless film that constantly forms on the teeth. The bacteria in dental plaque are what cause *periodontal disease*. If plaque is not removed carefully each day by brushing and flossing, it becomes calculus. In correctional environments where floss may be restricted due to security risks and concerns, alternative interdental devices will be provided. They include, but are not limited to: Soft Picks®, flossers, precut floss, Stimudents®, and proxy brushes.

Gingivitis: The first stage of *periodontal disease*. The gums usually become red and swollen, and bleed easily. This is brought on by the bacteria in *dental plaque* if it is not removed on a daily basis.

Implants: Artificial substitutes for tooth roots. Made from titanium and placed in the jaw, dental implants may be screw-shaped, cylindrical, or blade-like in form. Prosthetic teeth are attached to the part of the implant that protrudes through the gum. In many ways, dental implants function like natural teeth.

Maintenance therapy: An ongoing program designed to prevent *periodontal disease* from recurring in patients who have undergone periodontal treatment. It is also referred to as *supportive periodontal therapy*, formerly known as *recall.*

Root planing and scaling: A non-surgical procedure where the dentist removes *plaque* and *calculus* from the periodontal pocket around the tooth root and smooths the root surfaces to promote healing.

Supportive periodontal therapy: *Maintenance therapy* (see above).

2. Periodontal Disease Risk Management Protocol

The following BOP protocol is adapted from the *Oral Disease Risk Management Protocols in the Navy Military Health System*, BUMEDINST 6600.16A, August 23, 2010.

1) A Periodontal Disease Risk Evaluation may be performed on all BOP inmate dental patients during the comprehensive or periodic oral examination and recorded on the BOP form BP-618.060. Patients will be classified as low, moderate, or high risk for development of periodontal disease per the following risk factors.

   • **Community Periodontal Index of Treatment Needs Index (CPITN) Score:** Among clinical parameters, probing depths of 3.5 mm or more (CPITN 3 or 4) may be predictive of subsequent attachment loss. *Therefore, CPITN scores are the primary indicator of future periodontal diseases risk.*

   • **Tobacco use:** Smokers are four to five times more likely to have periodontal diseases than non-smokers. Spit tobacco use (sometimes referred to as smokeless tobacco) increases the risk of localized gingival recession, caries, and oral cancer.

   • **Genetic susceptibility:** This is assessed by asking the patient if any of his or her immediate family have lost teeth at an early age, have had treatment for periodontal disease, or have a history of diabetes.

   • **Oral hygiene:** Inadequate oral hygiene is predictive of gingivitis, and mild to moderate chronic periodontitis.

   • **Past history** of periodontal treatment increases the risk of future disease.

2) Determination of periodontal risk classification will prompt treatment protocols specific to the risk category. Required educational and treatment protocols for each periodontal risk category are summarized in *Table 3* below.

Table 3. BOP Protocol for Periodontal Diseases Risk Management

	Low Periodontal Risk	Moderate Periodontal Risk	High Periodontal Risk

Risk Criteria	1. CPITN 0, 1, or 2	1. CPITN 3, **plus** any *one* of the following:
		  a. Tobacco user
		  b. Inadequate oral hygiene
		  c. Family history of tooth loss or diabetes
		  d. Past history of periodontal treatment
			1. CPITN 4
			2. CPITN 3, **plus** any *two* of the following:
			  a. Tobacco user
			  b. Inadequate oral hygiene
			  c. Family history of tooth loss or diabetes
			  d. Past history of periodontal treatment

Protocol	1. Annual exam by general dentist and prophylaxis as needed	1. Annual exam by general dentist and prophylaxis by a dental hygienist 2. Recall schedule based on individual patient needs 3. Evaluation and discussion of periodontal disease risk factors	1. Annual exam by general dentist and prophylaxis by a dental hygienist 2. Referral for consultation to BOP periodontist (notify RDC) 3. Recall schedule based on individual patient needs 4. Evaluation and discussion of periodontal disease risk factors

3. Treatment Protocols for Various Clinical Diagnoses

The following recommendations are meant as guidelines to augment the clinician's judgment. See *Table 4* below for medications available on the BOP Formulary.

Chronic Periodontitis (Non-Surgical Treatment)

1) Thorough scaling and root planing; oral health instruction (OHI).

2) Reevaluation at 4–6 weeks (if problem areas remain, look for residual calculus or poor oral hygiene).

3) If generalized pockets persist:
   - Metronidazole (500mg) TID for 8 days, *or*
   - Doxycycline (100 mg) Q 12h on day 1, then 100 mg Q 24h for 21 days total

4) Supportive periodontal therapy.

Aggressive Periodontitis (Non-Surgical Treatment)

1) Thorough scaling and root planing; OHI concurrently with systemic antibiotics:
   - Amoxicillin (250 mg) *and* metronidazole (250 mg) TID for 7 days, *or*
   - Doxycycline (100 mg) Q 12h on day 1, then (100 mg) Q 24h for 21 days total, *or*
   - Metronidazole + ciprofloxacin (500mg) BID for 8 days of each drug

2) After antibiotics are used, continue with Periostat BID for 3 months.

3) Re-evaluate patient in 6 weeks to 3 months.

Diabetics and Smokers (Non-Surgical Treatment)

1) Treat as chronic or aggressive periodontitis, depending on your diagnosis.

2) If generalized pockets remain (following scaling and root planing) and systemic antibiotics are used, use doxycycline (100 mg) for 2 weeks as first choice; continue with Periostat for 3 months, and then reassess the patient.

3) During the supportive therapy phase, use local antibiotics for localized problems.

Table 4. Medications Available on 2012 BOP Formulary for Periodontal Disease Prevention and Management

	Medication	Directions
1	Alcohol-free Chlorhexidine	*Rx:* Swish 15ml of oral rinse undiluted for 30 seconds; then spit out. Use after breakfast and before bedtime, or use as prescribed. ***Note:*** *Despite medicinal taste, do not rinse with water immediately after use.*
2	Doxycycline (100mg)	*Rx:* Take 1 tablet q12h on day 1; then 1 tablet Q 24 hours for 21 days total.
3	Periostat (20mg)	*Rx:* Disp: 180 tablets; Sig: 1 tablet BID; Refills (2). Typically Periostat is prescribed for periods of no less than 3 months.
4	Amoxicillin (250 mg)	*Rx:* Take 1 tablet TID for 7 days.
5	Prevident 5000	*Rx:* Fluoride cream 1.1%; dispense 51gm of cream. Brush a small amount onto sensitive teeth at bedtime each night for 28 days; drink nothing for 1 hour following use.
6	Clindamycin (300mg)	*Rx:* Take 1 tablet TID for 8 days.
7	Metronidazole + ciprofloxacin (500mg)	*Rx:* Take 1 tablet BID for 8 days of each drug.
8	Metronidazole + amoxicillin (250mg)	*Rx:* Take 1 tablet TID 8 days of each drug.
9	Ciprofloxacin (500mg)	*Rx:* Take 1 tablet BID 8 days.
10	Metronidazole (500mg)	*Rx:* Take 1 tablet TID 8 days.

Dental Implant Maintenance

Although the reported long-term success rate for implants is good, it is important to monitor the patient and periodically evaluate and debride the implant. Maintenance intervals you choose may vary depending on the patient's ability to maintain the area. However, 6 months is the maximum maintenance interval, with 3 months being the average. Orton, et al. (1989) described the dental professional's role in implant monitoring and maintenance.

While it is important to document clinical parameters such as probing depth, clinical attachment level, bleeding on probing, and plaque and gingival indices, their prognostic value is currently unknown. It is important to note the following:

- **Progressive changes in probing depths** are more important than absolute depths.

- **Mobility** is a sign of implant failure.

- **Periodic radiographs** should be taken to evaluate for loss of implant integration (radiolucency) or excessive horizontal bone loss.

With Branemark fixtures, the mean horizontal bone loss during the first year is approximately 1 mm, and 0.1 mm/year thereafter (Albrektsson and Lekholm, 1989). Radiographs should be taken after the second-stage surgery at yearly intervals for the first 3 years to ensure proper fit of the abutment.

Removing Deposits from Dental Implants

When removing accretions from the implant, care must be taken not to damage the surface. Research shows that scratches on the titanium surface may result in increased plaque accumulation, corrosion, and a decrease in cell spreading (Fox, et al., 1990).

Rapley, et al. (1990) evaluated various instruments and materials to determine the surface changes produced in titanium abutments. The following instruments were evaluated: rubber cup, rubber cup with flour of pumice, air abrasive, interdental tapered brush, EVA yellow plastic tip, soft nylon toothbrush, universal plastic sealer, ultrasonic sealer, and a stainless steel sealer. Following instrumentation, the abutments were viewed with electron microscopy:

- Instrumentation with the interdental brush, EVA plastic tip, rubber cup, air abrasive, soft nylon toothbrush, or plastic sealer did not alter the implant surface.

- The rubber cup with the flour of pumice resulted in a smoother surface than the control.

- The air abrasive system produced a surface with dark discolorations, possibly indicative of surface corrosion.

- *Metal scalers appeared to gouge the titanium surface and produced significant vertical grooving. The air abrasive caused severe roughening, which was readily evident at the macroscopic level.*

These findings are in agreement with Fox, et al. (1990) who used a helium neon laser to evaluate implant roughness. Surfaces received 30 vertical strokes in a 2 mm area. Greater roughness was noted in surfaces treated with metal scalers (titanium curette > stainless steel) than those treated with plastic scalers or untreated controls (plastic scalers similar to control).

A subsequent study by the same group (Dmytryk, et al., 1990) reported cell attachment to be impaired in titanium surfaces scaled with metal instruments. The following hierarchy of fibroblast attachment was found: plastic curette > untreated control > titanium scaler > stainless steel scaler. This study suggests that other factors in addition to surface roughness may affect cell attachment since the titanium scaler that produced greater surface roughness than the stainless steel scaler did not affect cell attachment as much as the stainless steel scaler. In theory, metal scalers other than titanium cause corrosion, obliterating the titanium oxide surface layer and impairing cell attachment.

➜ *These results suggest that metal scalers and instruments such as ultrasonic scalers or the air abrasive __should not__ be used on titanium surfaces, since damage to the titanium-oxide surface will occur. However, plastic scalers and rubber cup polishing with flour of pumice will maintain or enhance the titanium implant surface.*

Oral Cancer Risk Assessment

Cancer of the oral cavity and pharynx accounts for approximately 3% of cancers diagnosed in United States (Nevelle, 2009). It is the eighth most common cancer in men and the fifteen most common cancer in females. Oral cancer rates are higher for black and Hispanic males, as compared to white males (American Cancer Society, 2011).

➜ *Health histories reveal that many inmates have risk factors associated with oral cancer. Understanding these risk factors is essential for all BOP health care providers. Early detection and intervention of oral cancers can save patient lives.*

The following BOP protocol is adapted in part from the *Oral Disease Risk Management Protocols in the Navy Military Health System*, BUMEDINST 6600.16A, August 23, 2010.

1) All inmate patients entering the BOP will have an Admission and Orientation Examination (A&O Exam) and a dental history in accordance with BOP Program Statement 6400.02. A soft tissue survey will be conducted. All dental staff should be familiar with the National Institute of Dental and Craniofacial Research (NIDCR) publication "Detecting Oral Cancer: A Guide for Health Care Professionals" (posted on Sallyport).

   Subsequent exams will be performed during Periodic and Comprehensive oral examinations and recorded on the BP Med 618. Patients may request an exam through dental sick call if they are concerned about a lesion that has been discovered or has not resolved. All patients will have a completed dental health history.

   Risk factors commonly associated with oral cancer are:
   - **Tobacco use:** Studies of oral cancer have consistently demonstrated that smoking and other uses of tobacco are the most consistently identified risk factors. Smokers have been found to have a 6-to-14 times greater risk of oral cancer compared to non-smokers.

The risk of oral cancer associated with smoking is equivalent for men and women, and diminishes with elapsed time since quitting.

- **Alcohol consumption:** Alcohol consumption is also a risk factor for oral cancer, especially with heavy consumption. The combination of heavy alcohol consumption with smoking increases the risk of oral cancer to a level greater than that resulting from either risk factor alone.

- **Age:** Oral cancer is closely related to increasing age, with over 80% of oral cancer deaths occurring in persons 55 years or older.

- **Human papillomavirus (HPV):** Patients exposed to HPV-16, a virus commonly associated with cervical cancer, have developed oral cancers. Oral cancers of a viral etiology, HPV-16, are typically seen in a younger cohort (< 50 yrs of age). These cancers are believed to be sexually transmitted (Oral Cancer Foundation).

- **Sun exposure:** Patients exposed to ultra violet rays from prolonged exposure to sun light are at a higher risk of developing carcinomas on the vermillion border. Day laborers and patients from Southern states are at a higher risk.

2) Determination of oral cancer risk classification will prompt treatment protocols specific to the risk category. Required educational and treatment protocols for each oral cancer risk category are summarized in *Table 5* below.

Table 5. BOP Protocol for Oral Cancer Risk Management

	Moderate Oral Cancer Risk	High Oral Cancer Risk
Risk Criteria	1. No lesions 2. One or more of the following risk factors: a. Tobacco use b. Moderate to heavy alcohol use (>2 drinks/day) c. Age 55 or older d. Exposed to HPV e. Excessive sun exposure	1. Presence of a potentially cancerous oral lesion
Protocol	1. Oral cancer risk education	1. Follow-up in 7–10 days; biopsy if not resolved 2. Oral cancer risk education

References

Albrektsson T, Lekholm U. Osseointegration: current state of the art. *DentClinNAm.* 1989;33:537–554.

American Cancer Society. *Cancer Facts & Figures 2011*. Atlanta, GA: American Cancer Society; 2011. Available at:
http://www.cancer.org/Research/CancerFactsFigures/CancerFactsFigures/cancer-facts-figures-2011

American Dental Association Council on Scientific Affairs. Professionally applied topical fluoride. Evidence-based clinical recommendations. *J Am Dent Assoc.* 2006;137:1151–1159.

Beltrán-Aguilar ED, Barker LK, Canto MT, et al. Surveillance for dental caries, dental sealants, tooth retention, edentulism, and enamel fluorosis – United States, 1988-1994 and 1999-2002. *MMWR.* 2005;54(30):1–44.

Beltrán-Aguilar ED, Goldstein JW, Lockwood SA. Fluoride varnishes. A review of their clinical use, cariostatic mechanism, efficacy and safety. *J Am Dent Assoc.* 2000;131(5):589–596.

Department of the Navy. *Oral Disease Risk Management Protocols in the Navy Military Health System.* BUMEDINST 6600.16A, August 23, 2010.

Dmytryk JJ, Fox SC, Moriarty JD. The effects of scaling titanium implant surfaces with metal and plastic instruments on cell attachment. *J Periodontol.* 1990:60:491–496.

Fox SC, Moriarty ID, Kusy RP. The effects of scaling a titanium implant surface with metal and plastic instruments: an in vitro study. *J Periodontol.* 1990;61:485-490.

Guerrero A, Griffiths GS, Nibali L, et al. Adjunctive benefits of systemic amoxicillin and metronidazole in non-surgical treatment of generalized aggressive periodontitis: a randomized placebo-controlled clinical trial. *J Clin Periodontol.* 2005;32:1096–1107.

Implants. In: *Periodontal Literature Reviews*, 1996:236–242. Available at:
http://www.joponline.org/toc/plr/current+volume/first+edition

Jenson L, Budenz AW, Featherstone JDB, Ramos-Gomez FJ, Spolsky VW, Young DA. Clinical protocols for caries management by risk assessment. *J Calif Dent Assoc.* 2007;35(10):714–723.

Marinho VCC, Higgins JPT, Logan S, Sheiham A. Fluoride varnishes for preventing dental caries in children and adolescents. *Cochrane Database of Systematic Reviews 2002*, Issue 1. Art.No.:CD002279.DOI:10.1002/14651858.CD002279.

Marinho VCC, Higgins, JPT, Sheiham A, Logan S. Combinations of topical fluoride (toothpastes, mouthrinses, gels, varnishes) versus single topical fluoride for preventing dental caries in children and adolescents. *Cochrane Database of Systematic Reviews 2004*, Issue 1. Art. No.:CD002781. DOI: 10.1002/14651858.CD002781.pub2.

Marinho VCC, Higgins JPT, Sheiham A, Logan S. One topical fluoride (toothpastes, or mouthrinses, or gels, or varnishes) versus another for preventing dental caries in children and adolescents. *Cochrane Database of Systematic Reviews 2004*, Issue 1. Art. No.:CD002780. DOI:10.1002/14651858.CD002780.pub2.

National Institute of Dental and Craniofacial Research (NIH). Detecting oral cancer: a guide for health care professionals. Available at: http://www.nidcr.nih.gov/OralHealth/Topics/OralCancer/DetectingOralCancer.htm. Accessed on September 13, 2011.

National Institutes of Health Consensus Development Panel. National Institutes of Health Consensus Development Conference Statement: diagnosis and management of dental caries throughout life, March 26-28, 2001. *J Am Dent Assoc.* 2001;132(8):1153–1161.

Nevelle, DA. *Oral and Maxillofacial Pathology.* St. Louis, MO: Saunders Elesvier, 2009.

Oral Cancer Foundation. The HPV connection. Available at: http://oralcancerfoundation.org/hpv/index.htm. Accessed on September 13, 2011.

Orton GS, Steele DL, Wolinsky LE. The dental professional's role in monitoring and maintenance of tissue-integrated prosthesis. *Int J Oral Maxillofac Implants.* 1989;4:305–310.

Rapley JW, Swan RH, Hallmon WW, Mills MP. The surface characteristics produced by various oral hygiene instruments and materials on titanium implant abutments. *Int J Oral Maxillofac Implants.* 1990;5:47–52.

Rethman MP, et al. Non-fluoride caries-preventive agents: executive summary of evidence-based clinical recommendations. *J Am Dent Assoc.* 2011;142(9):1065–1071.

Selwitz RH, Ismail AI, Pitts NB. Dental caries (seminar). *Lancet.* 2007;369(9555):51–59.

Slots J. Systemic antibiotics in periodontics. *J Periodontol.* 2004;75:1553–1565.

Suvan JE. Effectiveness of mechanical nonsurgical pocket therapy. *Periodontol 2000.* 2005;37:48–71.

Walsh T, Worthington HV, Glenny AM, Appelbe R, Marinho VCC, Shi X. Fluoride toothpastes of different concentrations for preventing dental caries in children and adolescents. *Cochrane Database of Systematic Reviews 2010*, Issue 1. Art. No.:CD007868.DOI:10.1002/14651858.CD007868.pub2.

Zero DT, Marinho VC, Phantumvanit P. Effective use of self-care fluoride administration in Asia. *Adv Dent Res.* 2012;24(1):16–21.

Attachments: Inmate Fact Sheets

The following Inmate Fact Sheets are attached for distribution:

- How to Reduce Your Risk of Tooth Decay

- How to Reduce Your Risk of Periodontal (Gum) Diseases

- About Your Oral Cancer Examination

These factsheets are adapted from:

Department of the Navy. *Oral Disease Risk Management Protocols in the Navy*. BUMEDINST 6600.16A, August 23, 2010.

Inmate Factsheet: How to Reduce Your Risk of Tooth Decay

Tooth decay ("dental caries") is caused by common bacteria (*S. mutans*) that nearly everyone has in their mouths. Two factors affect the ability of these bacteria to cause tooth decay—your diet and exposure to fluoride. Here are some important things you can do to help prevent cavities:

1. Reduce how often you eat or drink refined carbohydrates ("sugars").

- Tooth decay is affected by how many times a day you expose your teeth to refined carbohydrates. Whenever you eat, the bacteria in your mouth "eat" too. And when they do, they change the "sugars" in your mouth into an acid that attacks the enamel on your teeth. It takes about 20 minutes for the acid to clear from your mouth. So, every time you eat or drink something containing refined carbohydrates, your teeth are bathed in this acid for the next 20 minutes. The more time in a day that your teeth are exposed to the acid, the more likely it is that you will develop tooth decay.

- You cannot and should not eliminate all carbohydrates from your daily diet. Instead, try to reduce your number of between-meal snacks and limit your refined carbohydrate intake to mealtimes.

- If you drink soda (there are 12 teaspoons of sugar per can) or coffee with sugar, don't sip it over a period of time. This provides the bacteria with a continual supply of sugar! (Although diet sodas contain artificial sweeteners, they can still harm your teeth because they contain phosphoric acid.)

- Sweets aren't the only foods that promote acid formation and tooth decay. Many foods that people generally consider "healthy" (for example—fruit juices, sports drinks, and dried fruit like raisins) contain high levels of refined carbohydrates. Even salty snack foods such as potato chips, pretzels, and crackers (including saltines!) contain sugars that can lead to tooth decay.

- On the other hand, fresh fruits and many cheeses do not promote tooth decay, and are good choices for between-meal snacks.

2. Brush your teeth at least two times a day with fluoride toothpaste.

- Fluoride makes your teeth more resistant to decay. For maximum benefit, your teeth need frequent exposure to fluoride. Brush at least two times a day, for at least *two minutes* each time.

- Whenever possible, brush immediately after meals and snacks. This removes food particles and helps to clear the bacterial acids more quickly. Contrary to popular belief, rinsing with water after meals has very little effect on bacterial acids, although it may help clear away food debris.

- Always use a soft toothbrush, and floss your teeth at least once each day.

   In correctional settings, floss may be restricted due to security concerns. Alternative interdental devices will be provided to you such as Soft Picks®, flossers, precut floss, Stimudents®, or proxy brushes.

3. Use a fluoride mouth rinse at bedtime.

While you're asleep, you produce less saliva, leaving your teeth less protected from bacterial acids. Bedtime is the most beneficial time of day to expose your teeth to fluoride. So, just before you go to bed, after you've brushed and flossed, rinse with a 0.05% sodium fluoride rinse (Act® and Fluoriguard® are examples). Then, don't have anything else to eat or drink! This gives your teeth a "boost" of fluoride protection.

Inmate Factsheet: How to Reduce Your Risk of Periodontal (Gum) Diseases

The word "periodontal" literally means "around the tooth." Periodontal diseases are serious bacterial infections of the gum that destroy the tissue and bone that hold your teeth in place. Left untreated, gum disease can lead to tooth loss.

Periodontal disease is mainly caused by bacterial "plaque," a sticky, colorless film of germs that constantly forms on your teeth. In addition, if you have used tobacco, have diabetes, or have a close family member with periodontal disease, you are more likely to develop gum disease and possibly experience tooth loss.

Tobacco use:

- Smoking is considered one of the most important risk factors for periodontal disease, and spit tobacco use (smokeless tobacco) increases the risk of localized gum recession.

- While you no longer have access to tobacco products, it is important that you understand its effect on your dental health. You may already know that tobacco use is linked with many serious illnesses such as cancer, lung disease, and heart disease. You may not have realized that tobacco users are also are at increased risk for periodontal disease, even after they have stopped smoking.

- Smokers appear to be more likely to have serious periodontal disease, and less likely to respond to treatment than non-smoking periodontal patients. The probability of having periodontal disease increases with the amount smoked. However, the chances of having periodontal disease are lower in former smokers than in current smokers.

Diabetes mellitus:

- Diabetes is a disease that causes altered levels of sugar in the blood. If you are diabetic, you are at higher risk for developing infections, including periodontal diseases.

- The likelihood of periodontal disease increases when diabetes is poorly controlled, and can result in more severe gum disease than in non-diabetic patients. At the same time, infections such as gum disease can complicate the control of diabetes.

- For diabetics whose condition is controlled, periodontal disease responds well to treatment and can be managed successfully.

- It is important for the dentist to know if there is a history of diabetes in your family.

Genetic predisposition:

- There is strong evidence that heredity is a factor in the development of periodontal disease. If your parents or siblings have been treated for gum disease, or lost teeth due to gum disease, you may be at greater risk for this condition.

What you can do:

Your risk of developing periodontal disease increases with your number of risk factors. Of course, you can't change your heredity or that you have diabetes, but you can be aware of the risk they pose for gum disease, and take actions that optimize your periodontal health:

→ Follow your dentist's advice for maintaining good oral hygiene habits.

→ Reduce or discontinue tobacco use.

→ Follow your doctor's instructions for keeping your diabetes under control.

→ See your dentist regularly for examination and treatment.

Inmate Factsheet: About Your Oral Cancer Screening

Screening for oral cancer is an essential part of your regular dental check-up. Nearly 30,000 new cases of oral cancer are found every year in the United States. As with any type of cancer, the earlier it is found, the more successfully it can be treated.

Early detection is the key!

Early detection increases the chances of survival. All too often, oral cancers have reached an advanced stage by the time a patient seeks dental evaluation. Due largely to delayed diagnosis, the 5-year survival rate for oral cancer is only about 50%. However, oral cancer caught in the earliest stages has a much higher (85%) 5-year survival rate!

What are the risk factors?

- *Age:* The risk for oral cancer increases with age. The majority of oral cancers occur after age 40. As you get older, oral cancer screening becomes an increasingly important part of your dental exam. However, oral cancer can occur at any age.

- *Gender:* Males have nearly twice the risk of females.

- *Race:* African American males have nearly twice the risk of white males.

- *Behaviors:* Tobacco use (particularly smoking) and heavy alcohol use (more than 30 drinks per week) are associated with increased risk.

What you can do:

You have an important role in primary prevention and early detection:

- *Reduce your risk*: Avoid tobacco products and excessive alcohol use.

- *Don't wait*: In between dental check-ups, report any ulcer or sore in the mouth that does not heal within two weeks, or any unusual swelling in your mouth or neck.

- *Have regular dental check-ups:* Make sure to discuss with your dentist any concerns you might have.

Page Intentionally Left Blank

Page Intentionally Left Blank

Page Intentionally Left Blank